BURNING CANDLE

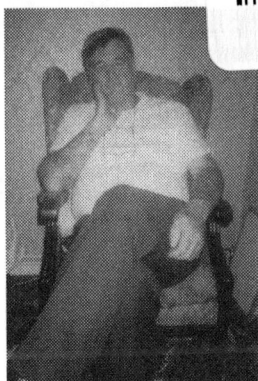

By Terry Beresford

"One million people commit suicide every year."
The World Health Organisation

Published by:
Chipmunkapublishing
PO Box 6872
Brentwood
Essex
CM13 1ZT
United Kingdom

http://www.chipmunkapublishing.com

Proof-read by Ben Vickers

ISBN 9781847471086

Foreword

It gives me a great deal of pleasure to be writing this foreword on behalf of Terry. I have known the author – Terry Beresford – for the past 10 years through my involvement with Basildon Mind. Terry was at that time already a Volunteer with the organisation in the role of Vice Chair and working on the Telephone Help Line.

It is a humbling experience having read so many of Terry's Poems that I feel I have been infused by his own personal journey with Manic Depression. Terry's Quest to help others has in turn, encouraged him to write with such enthusiasm and insight. Terry's Poetry is very powerful with extracts of flavour and real feeling that truly touches the reader's heart.

by Patricia Holdsworth BSc Hon.Dip. Counselling Manager Basildon Mind

Dedicated to my family and friends

15 Plus

Fifteen years, more perhaps,
My traumas have been rife,
Ten years on my wife, she says,
The demons spoilt the lot.
Attack, attack, day and night,
Enjoyment, look forward to!
Never felt that since '85 even more!
50th Anniversaries, retirement and awards,
I took with tears and strife; everything was flat, when I
was well!
Illness was a battle royal.
Me against the forces of evil,
Or so it seemed.
Now I rise, to rest and destroy the memory,
Of the evil that ruined all,
For all those years, family lived on a knife-edge.
Can't see, can feel it, hell!
Now I have secret to keep you at bay,
Write it down I say:-
I enjoy life from today
It's father's day.

50/50

Calls came in to stir the crews
Into gear, they swiftly dressed,
Machines at ready, the men mount up
Opening doors unleash these braves
They quickly head to fates unknown
Explosions heard, they near the scene
Engines turn and see the blaze
One is trapped, "save my child!"
A mother's cries are heard
Two don breathing sets
And into hell, they go.
Thick smoke no child to see
Fire, sweat it gets so hot
Give up "never" not these two
Backroom now a child is found
Snatched away to mother's breast
His partner still inside, but where?
Crews set up and start a search
A flash, as flames lick out the door
From within a blast is heard
Silence! From he who lagged behind
The air he breathes no more
Ultimate sacrifice has been made
A child will be a man
The brave one, an angel now
To guard and guide his kind.
Thanks dad.

1914-1918

A battle royal, oh no, not this,
Pure hell, sheer panic
The mud, the rain, the trenches deep.
Corpses lay in wait, so still
Gunfire blasts ears, one and all
No more will we see home
Families so far away.
In mist, they drift away.
The whistle blows and over we go
Cut down so fast, no time to run.
They barely cock their guns.
Bullets strike, sons and fathers fall.
Hung on wire, just bodies now.
Their souls have risen high
Left to rot and sink in mud
No burial for them, so sad.
Some lied and said their ages more.
Fourteen years boy and man, now gone.
Barely left his school desk and chair.
His name now etched in stone.
Remember them, they gave their all.
To save us from pure hell.
No way back, you went to die.
The few came home alone.
No hero's welcomed home.
Four years on and millions dead.

A MIND OF MY OWN

The Journey From Black Hole to Peacehaven

I could not rid myself of the awful feelings: - why not?
Muddled thoughts, weight loss, worry, hopelessness,
self Bereavement and loss. Full house! Alone in a
crowd I often felt, surrounded by friends and family,
threatened and remote, somehow different!

Doctors, therapists saw me, to no avail. Valium,
Librium, antidepressants to suppress my woes. Side
effects, they tell you not, pure hell, self-doubt, can
anyone see my suffering? No scars you see!

Memory loss, exhaustion, I struggle on, in the midst
of pure terror! Job loss, debt and pain, on it went,
deeper into the black mire.

More therapists, psychiatrists: - diagnosis, at last!
Overwork and stress, no more!

Unable to relax, gone too far, downhill downhill, living
in a box, unable to free myself. The flatness of life,
why go on?

No job, no hope, does no one understand? Can't
they help me? Please! In despair, no will to live, time
to go, the easy way out? Courageous or cowardly?
Please tell me, I want to do right, please tell me, I
know not!

Insane thoughts? Say nowt, they lock and drug you up, no fear! Not me, I'm a fighter, you'll not have me, get off my

back you evil black bastard, I'll fight you all the way, go away, you won't have me!

Battle commenced, the odds were high, could still be hell, win or lose! The road was long and treacherous.

I decreased the drugs, the pain increased, I went on and on, I cried, I prayed, I crawled, I pleaded, I died again and again!

NOTHING,

Doctors shouted and offered no aid, no time you see! I worked and struggled, my cloud now grey, albeit

a gathering storm within. Flashbacks, panic, nightmares, weird twisted extreme thoughts, life went on, I could not

cope, please let me get off! I cried and cried. A power inside possessed me, an automatic engine within, I felt good, I

felt high, I spent and spent, I drove, tankfulls disappeared – I went nowhere, round and round in circles, I talked, I

drank, bottles bought and consumed.

PANIC!! 999!! DOCTOR?? POLICE?? AMBULANCE?? HOSPITAL?? FIRE BRIGADE?? HELP??

ANYONE??....

I felt like a lowly animal, but why?

Illogical but logical in my twisted state, my clouded mind, was it 3-D? Unreal.

Home again, better, struggles on, try to hide it, that'll do! Didn't work, depression reared its cloaked head, stay in,

"DO IT!! DO IT!! GIVE EVERYONE SOME PEACE
AND DO IT.

YOU'RE A FAILURE!!"

Said a voice from the hole.
No way!! Get off my back!! Go!! I cried in pain. I was
losing. Release for a time, not long, to a manic stage,
no tiredness, felt strong as a lion, work all hours, I'm
superman, invincible, immortal. Worry? Not at all,
have a spend, that's good, but crazy, no sleep, non-
stop engine racing away, on and on and on…

PANIC!! 999!!
Away again. Burnt out. Twice more I went, a label at
last:

"MANIC DEPRESSIVE"

it said. "Relax", they said, a new word to me, I can't
do that - Medication removed, drugs ceased, the
replacement, the cure? A mineral salt? A rest, a
section, a prisoner, a wanderer, where to?
Cardboard city – sounds good to me, peace and
solitude, ALONE! But wait! What of the family? I
stay, for them. If they'll have me!!
Settling, therapy, tapes to hear, depression rife! So
bad. So high yet so low, without physical movement,
nowhere to go, unemployable, that's me. C.P.N.'s,
counselling, social workers, news to me, I'm not
insane!!
Still trod on, now bearable, understanding more.
Back to work? Not yet. "Try Mind", they said, I went,
it rained. I sat and thought, "What's this?" I wasn't
MAD! Why here? Warmth I felt indeed. Normal –
insane? Who was who? Can't see! Felt support,
heard laughter, no tears. I didn't want to stay, but
nowhere else to go now! Stay here and see!
Volunteer – that's it! That'll do! Sit 'round a table like
knights of old in Camelot'.
I felt needed, take on a task, they asked, I did.
Steady though, not too fast, the edge is not far away,
watch out, so steep, so dark, be wary.
Strived on, no fight or struggle, different now, not
alone. No friends lost, no one can see my scars,
confidence lifted my head, an animal no more, a man
of pride and upright stance, a friend, a diamond
amongst men, that's me!! I'm back, I think, no
doubting now. 'Feelgood Factor' in 5th gear, watch
overdrive, steady now, think of oneself, not too fast,

slow down or you'll rocket again, no sleep, be aware, it's a warning, take heed!! Verbal concerns must be noted, listen!! Take a break, don't get angry, relax. Help others, you can now that you're back, a Trojan from the war, sword in hand to battle once again, you know the way to slay the beast, that's beyond a doubt. Team spirit and support you have, you have him in the palm of your hand, the unseen DEMON cannot win. You're really back, it's Peacehaven and Mind is all around. Swords and guns not in this fight.

The warrior has his say:-

"We'll talk the bastard out!!"

he said:

"The demon within is now without! He's dead! REST IN HELL!!"

A SMITH'S JOURNEY

Terry joined the fireman's crew,
But felt all ill at ease.
He did so well, exams passed too!
He stayed on, as if to please.
No future here, with this fireman lot
Off he went to fortune find,
Reaching for his goals.
Day and night, work and work,
He really didn't mind.
Pitfalls, too many,
And dark, deep holes,
He rose above them all.
The empire grew and some good souls
Joined up and played the ball.
His roots remained intact, oh yes!
Friends and enemies he did make.
Head down, he strived, none the less,
Rewards were there for all to take.
Decision time, it must be read,
"Cut and run" the choice was clear
 "Pay and stay" the taxman pled!
To work so hard and pay that much
He could not 'cede to that.
To sell and fly, but keep in touch,
Would see him for a while.
Friends and family not far away,
You'll probably be home in May!

A SPIDER

Oh dear! I have a spider on my soul
He bites and nips for all his worth.
He's a nuisance from the black hole
Too much he nips and bites so, in his mirth
Perhaps he needs a swat or two
Nip is all he does
I'll slap him, that'll do.
Hell run away, with a cuss
Far, far away off he goes
To land on someone else.

ABSOLUTE BURN OUT

I'm dead, well nearly! Burnt out.
My heart pumping life's blood,
Remainder could be charred ashes,
But hey! What's this, no manic here,
Depression does not exist, too tired.
Sore feet, aching joints and muscles too!
No traumas of the mind
To stay in this state a little while
May just do the trick for me
Find a separate path footprints upon.
And pick up like phoenix bird
He rose, died, rose again and again.
That's exactly how I feel,
But this time dear, it must be here
To stay!
My head above!

ACES HIGH

They flew to save us from the Hun
So young, they had no fear
Wild and brave they steered their craft
To down the enemy threat.
Many died fighting the cause
Spinning and diving towards the earth
In flames they perished just ashes remain
No grave for these brave sons
Heavy hearts for those at home
A medal given for a life
Not wasted only missed
Boys were men the gallant "few"
They turned the tide from war to peace
"Thank you" we say, but no one hears
So sad.

ANIMAL, VEGETABLE OR MINERAL

Butterflies in my stomach
Lion in my heart
Cheetahs in my legs
My arms are ape like too!
Spine is of a giraffe
Towering high aloft
Roaming like a tiger
I swallow like a bird
I swan around all day
Or duck when the demon comes
I climb a little catlike
Barking mad like dogs too!

I grunt as pigs in clover
Sometime, I'm sheepish too
And all I know dear, is I just love you.

ARCHER QUESTION

Problems, I've had a few
Moans, groans, lots of them
Pain and anger, that too
Do not know from whence they stem
Highs and lows all around
No one seems to help
"Do the unthinkable" said a voice
"Ask the Archer"
"She will know, eventually"
I did too and it worked
Took twelve years to tally
I felt alive again.

BE FREE

A slave I was, to an ailment, so cruel
On top of the world in the morning
Down in the depths in the evening
Sleep, Sound some broken
Can't I be free! Yes free!
What have I done to deserve this?
I'm really getting fed up
I wanna be free, oh yes!
Bring forth the winner's cup
And then I'll be free
Oh yeah! We'll see!

BEHIND CLOSED DOORS

So Strong, he upright stands,
Look up to him, so proud he is,
Working hard, all hours god sent,
He tires and bends, too much, too long.
Weakening fast, tries carrying on,
No cry for help he gives,
Shaking, trembling – not thinking clear,
Hiding away, a place to weep.
Can't talk, no one will understand.
Help does come, in many ways.
A list too long to write,
Back now, he looks so strong.
His Achilles heel well hid.
Behind closed doors he suffers now,
And no one sees, not a soul!!
Oh no!!

BI-POLAR

Ying Yang, that's me, to and fro
 Up and down, poles apart
It's difficult as you can see
Jekyll and Hyde, rapid not slow
Oh, where, oh where is the key
To unlock my inner self,
And destroy it forever? It must go
From me forever, off my back
To live again would be a treat
That I may never meet
High too good, low so bad
I think at times I must be mad
Perhaps I am, mad that is
Insane, outsane, not a word!
But a feeling so strong!
It is!!

BILLY BOY

Billy cried all alone – Don't cry
All alone cried Billy boy – So alone
He'd wept and wept and wept – So sad
A world so cruel – So cruel
He thought he'd end it all – Goodbye
But why oh why – Who knows
Should he do such a thing?
Deserved not that at all – Not at all
Done no crime oh Billy boy
Just had a teacher – Mr. Pile
Billy's teacher is a paedophile.

BIRDS CRY

The birdie sang in sparrows herne
His lungs full of clean air
Can't sing as long as he used to
Pollution grows in his lungs, you see.
He's tired of coughing fits
He gently flies to warmer climes
Where pollution you can trust
It's milder and more bearable
Than here on the ole' 25 motorway, that is!

BLACK DAY FOR DANNY GRAY

The hole was there
My mates had gone
I called out to them all
Blooded and dazed, I saw a house
Amongst the blasted glades
A welcome here a drop of rum
I felt alone and ripped apart
Kind lady talked to me
Soldiers came to comfort and guard
Till "chopper" rotored in
"Take me home, away from this –
Eight best mates I've lost today-
This is my blackest day!

BLACK IS NOT THE COLOUR

CHURCH WAS HERE, I'D JUST MOVED IN,
SUNDAY T'WAS MY DAY TO THANK,
THE LORD FOR ALL MY BLESSINGS.
AS MAN AND BOY I ATTENDED TO PRAY,
BUT HERE THEY LIKED ME NOT,
THE PREACHER SAID, "GO, LEAVE THIS
PLACE",
MY CONGREGATION OBJECTS TO YOU.
YES! CHRISTIANS THEY ARE, BUT YOU,
YOU'RE BLACK, TOO MUCH FOR US TO BEAR.
SO GO "MY BROTHER" AND FIND A PLACE,
TO WORSHIP WITH YOUR FOLK.

BLIND MAN

Our sweet Lord, he made the world
It took him seven days
But looking down he was but dark
He raised arms above his head
And said "Let there be light
Earth, wind and fire, let's see what they will bring"
"One thing, for me, I'll put upon, my image"
Man, let's see how long he'll last
A predator, a genius, let's see for me
My son will take a look to see
He'll be alright, he'll not die
They will try to hang him up
Hidden amidst his kind
The meek shall inherit the earth
Or perish he deemed
So right this may prove to be
Materialistic man came, perhaps for just a while
"Money is the root of all evil"
"Remember my warnings" the Lord said, and left
For us to toil alone, to prove him wrong, we hope
Lust and greed did rule the earth; man was indeed a
cruel kind
Our Lord, he sent down rules, "commandments" he
said
"You must obey" – man must shun all mortal sins
Wars, battles, crusades, all in God's name
Man fought for land and riches
God did laugh so much, he was in stitches
Thinking man will only last 3,000 years from when his
son was hung.

BORDERLINE

I walk upon a razor's edge
To fall would see me past
Cautiously I walk the line
Forever I seemed to walk, can't last
I'll spin and drift away
Only to rise and try again
Trying's too hard now
I'd rather be slain in half
Or sitting in my favourite chair
By my fireside.

BORN TOO SOON

My God, I've had some silly ones,
Ideas that is, no more!
I thought one day, that man would fly,
Now that's a silly thought!
Travel miles in minutes too,
That's the best one yet,
Speak so clear across the world,
And watch live pictures too!!
Facts of life across the seven seas,
Oh no! I can't see that,
Cures for ills that maim and kill
A change of heart? Well, that's silly too.
In 1850, I was born,
I told my pals my tales,
That was it, my fate was sealed,
I lived behind locked doors,
"Mad as hell" they talked of me!
I wonder when they'll stop.
Soon I hope!
It's bedlam here!

BRAVEHEART

I wish I was a Scot!
And fought at Bannockburn
Many years ago!
With Wallace – William that be!
He died in agony – tortured,
Disembowelled, hung and drawn.
To rack his body went,
Ne'er did he submit – to mercy – no way!
Braveheart his name, brave his heart.
William Wallace 7ft tall, one and all.
Longshanks was his foe, an evil man
England was his domain – to rule, you see.
Better than the Scots, the English were,
Or so they thought, - the scum!
Quiet and peaceful, Scots so proud
"Freedom" called Wallace in death.
'Twas full of Scots that green land,
Much to Longshank's disgust.
Seduced the brides, taxed to hilt
The English bled them dry
Longshanks owed a lot.
Robert the Bruce, Prince Regent of Scots,
He battled alongside Wallace, oh yes!
But turned on him and did him harm
Treachery was rife to Bruce,
And Braveheart died because.
Victories were few and far.
Bruce, he turned again and fought the British too!
"Stand and be recognised!"

BROKEN ARROW

THE BEAST GIVES US FOOD, CLOTHING AND
TOOLS
THE PLAINS A PLACE TO LIVE IN PEACE
THE RIVERS QUENCH AND CLEANSE US ALL
AND GUIDES OUR HORSES HOME.
THE WHITE MAN CAME TO TAKE OUR LAND
BUFFALOES DROPPED SO FAST
A SPORT FOR THEM, SURVIVAL TO US
SOLDIERS, BLUE-COATS HARMED US SO
WHITE MAN HATED ALL OUR KIND
OUR WOMEN AND CHILDREN SUFFER
THEY CARE NOT WHO THEY HARM
TREATIES MADE AND BROKEN UP
BRAVES NO MORE WALK IN PEACE
THEY MUST STAY ON THE LAND
MAPPED OUT FOR THEM TO LIVE
NO RIGHTS AT ALL THE WHITE MAN GIVES
THE RED MAN'S DEMISE IS RIFE
NO MORE TO HUNT AND LIVE IN PEACE
GUNS AND SWORDS SEE TO THAT.

BUDS IN MAY

The flowers glisten in the morning dew
The sun raises its head, to shine so bright
Mother earth warms to its rays
And the bright moon goes to sleep.
Flowers beckon, their buds so tight
To open their scented heads.
The earth is in all its might
All plants now out of their beds
To colour and blossom for all to see
Nature will always shine through
Believe me it's true!

CALLED ELSEWHERE

Turmoil, trauma, tears a way of life
To a head it came and broke my soul
Bedlam, voices, nightmares too!!
Into care to clear my mind.
A path to tread, to heal my ills,
An open door, for all to see
To belong once more, a place to toil
Seven years past, my tasks complete
"Take up the pen" my mentors call
Move on, build no more
A haven now a town
Manned throughout, the best, we have
I gently drift to calmer seas
Burn no bridges, come back soon
They call to me; I heed and drop a tear
Maybe afar but always near.
Don't dismiss those ones so dear.

"CIVILISED BUTCHERS"

THE DANCERS COME, THEY CHANT AND SING,
DRUMMERS, PIPERS, THE WARRIORS CALL
RAIN, GHOST, SUN, THEY DANCE ALL DAY
WAR PAINT, BONNETS FOR ALL TO SEE
THEY DANCE TO HONOUR SPIRIT GODS
SPIRITS, BRAVES, ALL TRIBES COME NOW
WHITE MAN SEES ALL THIS,
AND SEES TO IT, NO MORE!!
CHRISTIAN RELIGION, THAT'S FOR YOU, LEST,
WE KILL, AND BURN YOUR HOMES,
NO TREATIES KEPT, NO TRUST IN MAN,
THEY HUNTED RED MAN OUT,
DESTROYED HIS CROPS, BUFFALO TOO!
THEY FLED TO PASTURES COLD
SOLDIERS CAME AND TOOK THEM BACK
TO LAND SET ASIDE FOR THEM.
SOME STAYED, STARVED AND DIED.
AMEN.

COMMUNICATION, GROWTH, FREEDOM

HE TOILED ALONE FOR MANY YEARS,
HIS THOUGHTS AS BLACK AS HELL,
NO ONE, BUT NO ONE COULD FEEL THIS BAD
THE END IS NEAR, SO MANY TEARS.
PANIC COMES, DEPRESSION TOO, HE 'S SO
VERY SAD.
AN OLD FRIEND CALLED TO CHAT ONE DAY.
HE UNDERSTOOD A LOT – THEY SAY,
OUR MAN UNLOADED ALL HIS FEARS
HIS SHOULDERS LIFTED HIGH.
DRAINED NOW OF ALL HIS THOUGHTS
HE FELT NOT ALONE, A COMFORT, THIS!
OCCASIONAL CHATS, A FRIEND HE COURTS,
NOW HIS LIFE RETURNS TO BLISS.
A MORAL HERE, SO SPEAK YOUR MIND AND
HAVE YOUR SAY.
WE'LL NOT TELL A SOUL,
TRY – FOR SURE, IT'LL "MAKE YOUR DAY"
WE ARE ONLY ONE OF A KIND.

CONFIDENTIAL MINDS

A broken soul enters once more
No hope, no will to carry on,
A welcome, an ear to listen to one,
Unload; feel free, a burden gone.
Flood all your fears away,
Advice is not within our grasp
Behind closed doors we heal
Strength begins to show its face
And confidence grows fast
Amid dark clouds the rays break through
Better now, one leaves our midst
Burdens left in another soul's ear
Happiness, contentment once lost,
Now back and all around
A soul arisen from below.

COOL RUNNINGS

HERE'S A MRS CHESNEY, ARCHER TO A FEW
SHE JOINED MIND A YEAR OR SO AGO
NOW THEY HAVE A QUEUE
ONE OF THE BEST IS MRS. C.
SAVED MY LIFE HER MERRY CROWD
NOW KEEPS ME ON THE RAILS
A FAMILY PLACE I COME AND GO
LOVELY PEOPLE, ONE AND ALL, THEY ARE A
SIGHT TO SEE
IN DEPRESSION, I NOW NEED HELP
IN MANIC, I CAN ENJOY SO MUCH
IN A FUNNY SORTA WAY
THE HIGHS AND LOWS OF LIFE
COST ME LOTS OF STRIFE
STILL, I DON'T MIND – HONEST, MY LIFE

CORNED BEEF

HAVE YOU TRIED THIS STUFF,
SOME SAY IT'S PRETTY ROUGH.
BITS OF MEAT, FAT, GRISTLE TOO,
BULLY BEEF 'TWAS NAMED, WAY BACK.
SUSTAINED OUR WARRIORS IN THE WAR
SO IT CAN'T BE ALL THAT BAD,
IN A SARNY – BRANSTON TOO!
YOU'D MARCH ON A FULL TUM,
BUT WATCH YOURSELF, SOLDIER BOY,
HAS FIBRE MIXED IN TOO!
EAT TOO MUCH AND YOU WILL SEE
THE LOO A TIME OR TWO!!
WHOOPS!!
PARDON MEEEE!!!

CYCLES

You are here!.

The seed of life drops in the earth
It warms and thrives unseen.
Roots and shoots in abundance
The power within grows strong.
Green leaves begin to show
The sun and rain assist the growth
Upwards, upwards, towards the sky
With buds now open.
The cycle complete – a flower
Yellow, gold, red, perfume too!
Dropped leaves and wilted now
'Tis the beginning of the end.
Brown petals and decay now form
All returns to ground
Till spring of course
And you'll return to please us once again

DEPTHS OF

The demon within destroys, unseen,
The joker of despair,
He breaks you down, no pity,
No mercy his motto,
Uncaring, no feeling,
Cutting you apart, hidden from all
Medication he loves, they weaken the soul.

Down, down to his black lake,
Tormentor of the mind,
Lucifer is the name?
Fight him all the way, push back,
He'll weaken in the end.
Talk him out, he hates that,
Share him, he weakens.

Now in the open, he cannot work,
His demon tools now blunt.
He's in the light, he cannot see,
He suffers now,
Searching for another weak soul,
Gone from you, that's good,
Battles lost, but the war is won.

DEVIL'S DIG

The Devil's Dyke is deep 'tis true
It stretches far and wide
Was it nature formed this land
Or disciples toiling hard.

Dig and shovel day and night
The mounds and hills built up though
The Devil did little to clear the plains
He sat and sang a song
So bad it was, the workers fled
The Dyke was not complete.
His demons, they did finish off
And the Devil felt full of glee.
The Devil's Dyke 'twas now a place
To roam or fly a kite
Beware the Devil he's all about
To set tasks for you all.

DILDOUGH???

What is a dildough?
Not in any books to see!!
Can you cook with it??
Or is it to wear?
Never seen one
Only heard the name
Some laugh when I ask
It's not funny
I want one
Perhaps, one day
I'll get hold of my own
Then I can decide
On it's use for me!!
So – What is a dildough??

DON'T QUIT!

The will to win
A fight, battle on a race
Ill prepared is failure be
"Practice makes perfect" so they say
To fly, swim or run
Higher, stronger, faster
The goal in hand is hard
To fail is unacceptable
Second an "also ran"
The winner goes down in history
Immortal to us all
Gold on stone, forever carved
Keep going I say what ere your goal
You'll come through were sure of that
Dedication, that's the word
And a will to win.

EASE TENDERS

Nine years I toiled
For Mind alone
Soon to rise like the phoenix
From the fires Ashes too
Next time to mend my ways
Fifteen years of turmoil
The Lord? He owes me now't!
A family made, children too!
At home and away at Mind
They came, they saw, they conquered
A fireman gone, with more to come
Soldiers guard and police my mind
So I can be free as a bird
A dove, I'll be and write a book.

ENLIGHTENED

I CHANGED MY TASK
'TWAS ON MY MIND
SEVEN YEARS ON
A JOB WAS FORMED
TOO MUCH TO CARRY FOR TOO LONG
MY SANCTUARY IS NOW MY DEN.
I WRITE AND PLAY MUSIC A LOT
MY SPIRITS RESTORED, NOTHING TO DO.
I FEEL IT'S WASHED FROM ME.
I DO AS I PLEASE EACH DAY
CAN I NOW BE LEFT ALONE?
TO CARRY ON AND FINISH OFF MY TASKS
SET FOR ME TO DO
NOT MUCH, ENOUGH! I SAY TO YOU,
NEAR 20 YEARS THAT FEELING STAYED,
CONTROLLED NOW, HELD AT BAY,
SHARE IT OUT NO MORE!!

EVERYONE IS HELPING ME

Everyone is helping me
Yes they are
Like an army
I am surrounded
To keep demons out
Sometimes they get to me
But not for long
They depart – flee
And make me feel
A man alive again
A slave to him I was
That devil in disguise
Tormentor, now wait outside
I'll see you when I'm ready
On my terms, that is
Thank you my little helpers
You're diamonds, truly.

FINAL CUT

BROKEN CIRCLE, IT HAD COME,
CAUGHT AT WOUNDED KNEE,
OLD WARRIORS, WOMEN, THE CHILDREN TOO!
SABRES SLICED THEM ALL.
BULLETS FLY, WE DROP LIKE STONE,
THEY'RE HERE TO KILL US ALL,
NO MORE TO RIDE AND HUNT IN PEACE
THIS BEING WANTS THE LOT,
OUR INJURED TAKEN BACK TO TOWN,
IT'S SNOWING AND CHRISTMAS TIME,
A SINGLE BANNER BLEW IN THE WIND,
PROCLAIMING "PEACE AND GOODWILL TO ALL
MEN"
RED MAN WAS NO MORE!

FIRE OF DOVES

Wings that whistle in the dark
Flames that burn so bright
Feathers blown along the ground
As doves fly off in peace
Escaping fury of the fires
Their tails and feathers singed
More feathers in the sky
Now they gather in their cote
To flap their wings and "Coo" to you
That's their haven
Peacehaven
no more

FIREBRAVES ARE A COMING

For all to see and hear
They put out flames
Save lives too – plus a risk or two
Fire braves they are the best
In towns and villages too
One life saved is worth all the gold
Snatched from the devils claw
By fire braves, nothing better
To live life to fulfilment
You know that makes sense
Fire braves stand alone – Elite!
Southwark trained, London men, the cherry on the cake
But everyone knows that
True tradition, the name of the game
True grit is their middle name.
By Christ! They are so brave
None will ever surpass
Fire and water is their skill
Either one can surely kill
No one can surpass
The skill of the fire braves
Hard as nails soft as mud
You may think, but think on
When in trouble, who's called out
A shout a cry for help
Up and at 'em, that's the way
A cry for help they cannot refuse
The fire braves – The crème de la crème forever.

FOOTLOOSE AND FANCY FREE?

Do you know what it's like?
When you've forgotten how happiness feels?
Oh! To be happy, content every day.
I have just realised after 20 years
I'm stricken with being flat, then low,
When high I know I'm ill, so sad
True happiness now beyond my reach.
Yes, I laugh and joke with most,
But I turn around and tears may roll
Only tiredness drops my shield
It can be seen by those who know
Others look forward to this and that
With me, I await judgement day
When I can rest in peace
The sooner the better
Believe me; enough's enough.

FOOTPRINTS TO SERENITY

I cannot change this way of life
So fraught with ups and downs
I fought and died so many times
Knew not where to turn
A 'Don' came to me to comfort my trauma'd mind
He softly said, "Go to Mind".
Mad I thought! I have a mind
Albeit all mashed up
No! Mind to rest and Peacehaven
The footprints in the sand he said
Nine long years a minder now
Felt 'twas time to rest
So much done we have to keep mum
No one would believe our goal!
So there!

FOREVER CAPTIVE

I SIT HERE NOW, ALONE, NOT A CARE,
THE WORLD RUSHES ON AND ON, SO FAST!
SHOOTING, KILLING, STARVATION TOO!
BASIC HUMAN RIGHTS ARE RAPED
BY DICTATORS HARD AND CRUEL.
BULLIES NEED TO BE CUT DOWN
THEIR WORK IS SATAN'S JOY!
COWARDS THEY ARE, BEHIND A SHIELD
REAL HEROES OPPOSE THEIR REGIME.
FREEDOM FIGHTERS NEVER DIE,
THEIR CAUSE GOES AHEAD, SO TRUE.
DRUG BARONS, PAEDOPHILES, WE HATE,
JUSTICE? THEY ESCAPE, DOWN HERE ON
EARTH,
GOD RUBS HIS HAND WITH GLEE.
HIS JUSTICE IS ETERNAL, NO END.
THIS SCUM WILL PASS TO HELL.
FOR LIFE? NO, FOR DEATH, ETERNITY!
WHOOPEE!

FULL CIRCLE

Life is but a mirage
An Oasis all around
Heartbeat stops, your game is done
Another steps in to play
Problems, problems, we make them all,
A circus act, we have not long.
Eternity that be changes not,
Weight of the world on his back,
Stress will see a scrambled mind,
Centuries come and centuries go,
So trivial, worry not on this.
The oasis waits for one and all,
Pollution fades away, so slow,
Now man has fled this mother earth,
She can breathe again. Thank God.

GAME OF LIFE

OH, THESE MEN, WHO COUNTRIES RUN,

THEY THINK IT IS A GAME

IN THE DARK THEY STUMBLE ON,
ONES OPINION CAN START A WAR,
SQUEAKY CLEAN, RACIST PIGS,
TERRORISTS, KILLERS, NOW AT THE HELM
I.R.A., U.D.A., ALL FEEL THEY ARE RIGHT,
SADDAM, ARAPHAT HAVE SHADES OF DOUBT,
THEY LEAD OR BULLY TO HAVE THEIR WAY,
CHRISTIAN, MUSLIM, EVEN WORSE,
FIGHTING LIKE CAT AND DOG,
FOR WHAT, POWER? CASH OR LAND?
LEADERS TALK ALL AROUND THE WORLD
WHY CAN'T WE CEASE AND HELP.
CHILDREN DIE, NO FOOD TO EAT,
JUST GRAINS UPON THE DIRT,
PAINS OF HUNGER WE'VE NEVER HAD,
CAN'T WE GIVE SOME MORE
RED DICTATORS – WIPE THEM OUT,
LET'S BALANCE UP THE SCALES.
IF NOT HERE UPON THIS EARTH.
THE COURT OF HEAVEN STANDS,
YOUR JUDGEMENT COMES IN DEATH.
LIFE IS BUT A MIRAGE.

GLAD AND SAD

Winter comes, we are sad
Summer here we are glad
Raindrops on our face
The sun within your heart
Go with the flow, at your pace
Stick with nature, don't grow apart
Butterflies, they come and go
Buds flower, they have made a start
Birds duck and dive in the skies
Bees and wasps fly around the flowers
Pollinating and feeding all day
It comes and goes, glad and sad
Sit down; relax in sun's warm rays
Imagine the sun is all around for days
No winter in your heart.

GO WITH THE FLOW

It came upon me in a different way,
It ripped my guts away
Damage done, for all to see,
So powerful, fearful, just not me.
Perhaps next time I'll kill
No way – not on – time to change
It caught me out, no time to run,
But my memory stays intact.
To recall, Assess and plan defeat
Return the compliment that's what I'll do
Surprise, Change tack, beat the bum,
Fight, keep on, it'll soon come.
Albeit a different way.
Boundaries 'amust, to save defeat
Others must guide me though.
If we are to gain our goal
In cotton wool I'll win the war,
Is that a lot to ask?
Prove myself, no need for me
An open book I feel.
Slow down, take nothing on

GOING TO THE DOGS

Oh sister dear, I have a fear
It's money down the drain, no less,
Traps one to six, oh what a fix,
The form, the odds, the silly sods
They know not head from tail.
Winners, losers, join the club,
Friday comes, you'll need a sub
Have a drink, a bite to eat,
Tote is open, bookies to beat
Second last race! – it's 9.30
A fiver? Bus fare home!
Honour Cheryl, A lively bitch,
Let's put it on, I'll have to hitch
In hot pursuit my dog leads,
It takes them all by storm,
Quids in now! A slap up feast,
Chicken legs and diet coke, oh no!
A Chinese, A drink and a bone for the beast!

GOLD RUN

Years of training for a gold,
Now within your sight,
Starter's gun the stories told
Push, run, with all your might,
In the lead at half-way mark
You feel you're steering clear
Maybe a trick, a mindless lark
To stop your winning way
To win you must, it is so dear,
Total dedication it must pay
Goal in sight, so close and near
You're over in first place
A gold! At last, for all to see
And it's just another race.

GREEN-PEACE

EARTH, FIRE AND WATER,
MAN MAKES A LOT FROM THAT
GREED AND MONEY HAND IN HAND,
WE REALLY DIDN'T OUGHT'ER
CUT TREES AND FLOOD THE LAND
GOD'S CREATURES STARVE AND DROWN
EAT YOUR MONEY, THAT DAY WILL COME
"NATURE CANNOT BE BEAT" SAY SOME
FIRE AND FLOOD WILL SEE TO THAT
SHE WASHES HER HANDS OF US
POLLUTION CLEANSED, SIMPLE; NO FUSS!
IT MUST BE GOOD FOR ALL,
WE TAKE TOO MUCH NOW COMES A FALL,
MOTHER EARTH RECLAIMS - AND SOON!
GREEN GRASS, FRESH AIR, THE SUN AND
MOON,
SOUNDS GOOD TO US, SO COME ON DOWN.

GROUND ZERO

Planes in the skies
Crashed into towers aloft
The fuel ran out so fast
Ignition saw the building burn
People jumped to no avail
Panic all around and on the ground
One tower collapsed, killing all
Fire-fighters, rescuers too
All buried beneath
That tower so high
Tower two groaned and went
Deep into ground zero
Many killed in this devilish deed
"Terrorists" they say, "let's get them"
Trouble is – get one, and others come to the fore
They terrorise the whole world
It really is the third world war
So sad, so true.

HAPPINESS! WHAT'S THAT?

I'm bored stiff at times
Can't remember lasting happiness
It's disappeared from my mind
I can't recall at all
I laugh and joke to all around
It's mostly tears of the clown.
My feelings mostly low and flat
"Cheer up pal" I wish I could
A low life, is what I feel.
No lift on excitement here,
When high, I know I'm ill,
When low it is pure hell,
Middle be flat, no more.
Constant feelings up and down
I'm really getting sick
And tired of this rotten life,
I think I'll end it soon.

HELL E COPTER

The grim reaper cometh on the wing,
His blades did slice 100ft up.
It was hell for all inside
Two reapers had struck
It was the Holocaust
Not nature's wrath,
Mans – Hatred to other men.
Down they came to ground zero
Tumbledown, the bricks and dust
People ran – though too slow
To die and rest in peace
Many lived, only to die
Under tons of bricks and rubble
Whoever did this is in real trouble!

HERE TO STAY

MAN'S CONCRETE CRACKS AS NATURE SHOWS
WE'RE FIRMLY IN HER GRASP
CEMENT OR TAR, THE GRASS STILL GROWS,
MAN REPAIRS AND COVERS, MAKES AND
MENDS.
"PROGRESS" MAN SAYS, HE'S RICH AND FAT,
MOTHER EARTH WILL OVERCOME, NO FEAR.
THE DAYS ARE FEW FOR MATERIAL MAN,
NATURE WILL NOT BE SUPPRESSED,
SPIRITUAL MAN HAS ALWAYS BEEN,
HE'S GONE ALONG, WITH HEAD IN HANDS,
A TEAR RUNS DOWN HIS FACE.
GREED, MONEY, POLLUTION, CANNOT MAN
SEE?
THE GRAVE TAKES NO CHEQUES, CARDS OR
CASH
PHARAOHS RICHES DO NOT RETURN,
THEY REMAIN IN COLD STILL VAULTS, DEAD!
MODERN MAN WANTS THE LOT, NOT ALL,
JUST SOME WITH SPIRITS WANED,
BUT HEED THESE WORDS AND THINK AWHILE,
OIL AND FUEL WILL BE CONSUMED,
WE TOIL SO HARD TO PRODUCE ALL THIS
YET NATURE HAS IT ALL, JUST FOR US,
TAKE FROM HER WHAT YOU NEED, NO MORE!
THE BUFFALO DIED, BUT TRIBES REMAIN.

HILL TOO FAR

The road was narrow
The trees were high
Soldiers in formation passed by
Guns glaring in the late sun
Six good men, troopers too
Walking on the path to hell
A click! All stop – take cover
Bushes here, bushes there
The sniper fires from anywhere.
One goes down, shots are heard
Someone screams beneath a bush
A soldier fires, it stops
Rustling in the thicket
The enemies on the run
Troopers move in for the kill
Injured, dead, not one remained
Upon this hill too far.

HOME FROM HOME

Home from home, that's what it is
To come and go as I please
Friendly faces, no threat, the biz!
Have a cuppa, a cake or roll
You can even get out and have a stroll
Laurie, Pat, Sheila, Peter, just a few
A lifesaver it was for me, so true!
Oh yes! A real lifesaver – for me
So one and all, you must see
It helped me, I helped others
Like a family – sisters and brothers
That's where I belong!
So there I'll be.

HOMEWARD HEROES

RAGING GUNS, THE BOSUN CALLS
SAILS CRASHING TO THE DECK
EXPLOSIONS BLAST THE CREW
GUNPOWDER SMELLS, SMOKE DRIFTS AROUND
THE CAPTAIN LIES IN BLOOD
HIT BATTLE WON BUT LOST
ENEMY DRIFT AWAY FROM US
STINGING WITH DEFEAT
WINNERS, MAYBE, BUT LOSSES GREAT
TO FIGHT ANOTHER DAY, A FEW.
AS HEROES DOCK AND CROWDS DO GREET
THE FLEET LOST 6 FROM 12
DRY LAND AFFORDS OUR TIRED SOULS
OUR THOUGHTS AWAY AND BODIES HOME.

I'M IN AN AWFUL WAY

Oh dear! I've got a headache
My leg is sore too
My neck's rather stiff
I have a sore toe
My mind is in a mess
Back is aching so much
Eyes ache, no sleep
Oh dear, oh dear
My heart is strong
I have heartburn
I'm in a state
My joints all ache
I've a sore finger
Writer's cramp too
Still, I accept all my woes
I'll not complain any more
Today.

I WHISPER IN THE MORNING

I whisper in the morning
My head is dull, near dead
"Arise my son" The Lord he said
I find it hard to obey
But do it to save face
Demons, demons in my head
Too much, too much
I've to pace myself
The demons in my thoughts
I've tried lots and lots
To defeat the horrors
Within my brain, oh yes!
They come and go, too much for me
I'll do myself in
Ha! Ha! Or will I? We'll see.
You demon of my mind
"Wanna fight?"

IF IN DOUBT ACT STUPID

DO YOU KNOW WHAT THAT CHEEKY SOD SAID?
THE DEVIL THAT IS THE LEADER OF MY HELL,
HE SAID TO ME: "IF THOUST WISHES TO BE
FREE OF THESE MIND TRAUMAS"
OBVIOUS! I THOUGHT!
"THEE MUST LIVE A LIFE IN PENANCE OF ME!"
"GET STUFFED", I UTTERED
"TO FIDGET AND FLY AROUND IS WHAT I
DREAM"
 I COULDN'T BELIEVE MY EARS
I'VE DONE JUST THAT FOR YEARS,
"TO NE'ER REST, BUT KEEP TO TOIL,
FOR ETERNITY – OF COURSE!!
"Y-YES PLEASE DEVIL, I'LL DO ANYTHING"
I GASPED
WHAT A PRAT, I THOUGHT.
HE DID JUST THAT AND NOW I'M FREE
FOR ETERNITY!

IN MY EYES

Look into my eyes
You'll not see
All I have, within my eyes
Demons, dreamscapes, nightmares
Only for me to see
So hard for me
No others can see
No broken arm or fractured leg
Yes I'm ill, you see it not
God only knows
Apart from me
Highs and lows
He's with me all the way
Each and every day
The horrors of black hole
The elation of manic
So cool, forever.

IN THE BEGINNING

SETTLE DOWN, ENJOY THE CALM
YOU CANNOT CHANGE THE WORLD,
MAN, AS A WHOLE, IS DOING SO,
POLLUTION, GREED, CORRUPTION, MONEY,
ALL DO TAKE THEIR TOLL,
MOTHER EARTH CAN SEE ALL THIS
OUR TIME MUST BE NEAR OUT,
RESOURCES ARE APLENTY NOW,
LIKE TIN, THEY'LL DRY UP SOON
AN AGE TO MAN IS BUT A SIGH
HIS TIME HAS CAUSED A RIFT,
PROFIT AND GAIN, HE SEES NO MORE,
WEATHER CHANGES, ACID RAIN,
UNHEEDED WARNINGS FOR ONE AND ALL,
WILL EARTH GROW HOT AND BLOW AWAY,
OR CAN MAN RETURN TO EDEN,
WHERE IT ALL BEGAN.
WE'LL SEE!!

IN THE MIDDLE

Old Tel was on his last, or so the devil thought
"Oh Beelzebub" the Almighty said "'Tis only doing as he's taught!
"He's mine" the devil said, "He finishes unto me"
God did smile as he thought on, with a little glee
But Tel didn't know what God had said
He'd forgotten you see and was nearly dead
But he fought against those in mind
Befitting he would die he thought, than be a cowardly kind
Demons mash his brains to pulp "When will he die?" They called aloud
By his own hand this one must go
All sons of the devil must die this way
They cannot go, they must stay
Stuck in the middle they be
He'll not know who's telling him
Live, and it will be over
Die and it will be over
That's the way it is for him
He's truly a son of God, he lives!!
The devil scorned his demons
But unlike God, the devil had no footprints
He could never win.

IN THE SHADE

TWO SIDES, ONE DARK, ONE LIGHT, FOR ALL
TO SEE.
THE DARKEST IS TO FEAR,
THE LIGHT FOR ALL TO SEE.
THE DARKEST IS THE HORROR FACE,
THE LIGHT FOR ALL TO SEE.
IN DARKNESS, REVENGE IS UPPERMOST
THE LIGHT FOR ALL TO SEE.
DARK SIDES NEVER SEEN BY US,
THE LIGHT MAKES SURE OF THAT.
JECKYLL AND HYDE, BATS FROM HELL,
A MYSTERY OF LIFE.
WE ALL POSSESS THE PAIR OF THEM,
THE DARKNESS AND THE LIGHT.

INNERMOST GRIEF

Titanic strength is not enough
To counter the evil within
It darkens all hours – too much!
To leave and my spirits lift
A change of mood, that's all,
To confuse and flatten on its return,
I know not where to next.
Manic – depression, the pain is great
Legs, back, now shoulders too
They weaken under my mind's load.
Longer spells of ills come now
"'Tis me who's torn in half!"
Poles apart my feelings are,
My mind now starts to blur.
Days go by, my door is shut,
Contentment ne'er knocks or calls.
Please God, seek my tormentor,
Lock it up and throw the key,
Lord, - keep it away from me,
Words cannot tell my pleas,

IT'S ALL IN THE MIND

I sit here in peace
The sun shines upon my face
Winds be soft and gentle
Calm comes over me, no harm
Methinks the demons have gone
So quietly I speak and carry on
Perhaps he thinks I'm dead
For he had gone from my head
Time being anyhow
His deadly traumas have now ceased
The deadly demon holds back his beast
Perhaps now, yes! Now, I can live without
These traumas of the mind.

JACK AND JILL

Jack and Jill
Ran the corner shop
Both happy and smiling
They were – The best, simply
All shoppers loved them
Plunderers came, one morn
They robbed them at gunpoint
"Nothing" said Jack, "Give them nothing"
Jill tried to run
From the one that had the gun
He fire, Jack fell down
And broke his crown
And Jill came tumbling after
They called the police
As injuries allowed
Police arrived
Too late, both were no more
Struck down by thugs
For a few pounds
Money is the root of all evil.

KIPPERS 'N' CUSTARD

SHAKY BILL WOULD CUT OUR HAIR,
HE'D NIP AND CUT OUR NECKS.
SNIP A SLICE FROM OUR EARS,
HAIRCUT TIME, OH NO – ME DEARS!!
THE DEMON BARBER?
NO! NOT BILL.
HE HAD THE SHAKES AND TRIMMED OUR HAIR.
ONE STYLE – SHORT, BACK AND SIDES.
5P HIS PRICE – A SHILLING THEN.
AS HE CUT, HIS TONGUE WOULD DART IN AND
OUT HIS MOUTH.
THE ONLY BARBER IN THE TOWN
HOBSON'S CHOICE IT WAS, OH YES.
OUR VISITS TO OLD SHAKY BILL.
WE'LL NEVER FORGET!

LAST THOUGHTS OF THE DAMNED?

FROM PRISON CELL, THEY CALLED MY NAME,
THE PREACHER CAME INSIDE,
HE BLESSED ME ONCE AND ONCE AGAIN,
I ROSE TO FACT MY FATE,
A SHORT WALK NOW, TO OPEN DOORS,
THE GOVERNOR WITH TWO SCREWS CAME
TOO.
ALL SET TO WATCH ME DROP,
"INNOCENT" I SAID TO ALL, SOME ASKED FOR
CLEMENCY.
NONE GIVEN, MORE'S THE PITY, I'M GUILTY
THAT'S THE TRUTH
KILLED THEM ALL AND TORCHED THE PLACE,
THEN KILLED AND KILLED AGAIN.
HALTING AT THE DAUNTING SIGHT
THE STEPS LED UP TO HELL.
SHOVE ME, PUSH ME, THAT'S WHAT THEY DID,
I STOOD NOW, ATOP OF TRAP,
A NOOSE ABOVE MY HEAD,
DARKNESS FELL, A MASK PUT ON,
THE PREACHER SAID HIS BIT,
MY HANDS AND FEET, TIED SO TIGHT,
I WAITED FOR MY FATE,
ROPE PUT ROUND MY NECK,
JUST A DROP AND THEN A TUG,
MY NECK WAS STRANGLED HARD,
SO BLACK, I WONDERED HOW LONG NOW,
BEFORE MY MAKER COMETH.

LIFE IN CIRCLES

Round and round, that's how I go
No physical movement anywhere
Round and round that turns so slow
Circles of life, no one seems to care
Times are, when I spin like a top
Others send me to black hole
All this really must stop
Or else I'll call the day
I cannot stand much more
It's like living on a pole
Up, down, holding on, please, no more
But who's left if I do me in?
A family, each with cares for me
It would break them. They care you see.

LIFE OF RILEY

SCRATCH, SCRATCH, TEARS AND RIPS,
EVERYWHERE YOU'LL FIND THEM, FAST
ASLEEP.
FU N TIME COMES AND GAMES TO PLAY.
JUMPING, BITING, KICK BOXING TOO.
TINS ARE OPENED, A SMELL OF FOOD,
HEAD FOR KITCHEN, DON'T BE LAST.
LOTS OF GRUB, FRESH MILK TOO,
OUT WE GO FOR A NICE POO!
BACK AGAIN TO SETTLE DOWN
GET IN EARLY, GRAB YOUR PLACE
SNUGGLE DOWN TO WATCH TV
HECTIC DAYS ALL CATS AGREE.
WHAT SAY YOU?
MEOW!

LIFT YOUR HEAD

Come on sweet child
Lift your head
For all to see
Don't cry, no tears to shed
Relax, lie back – there's no fee
Too long you've run away
Helping other souls in doubt
Give up, you are done
Don't speed or shout
Please no – no more
For God's sake he knows
Slow down, before you burn out
Retire, rest, all is done
Relax! Forever,
And lift your head.

LOST AND FOUNDED

My heart so keen, my mind so meek
I'll need to rest a while at times.
But giving up is not for me
I'll back you all the way.
So, go for it sister dear.
My sword is raised and charged.
My strength restored for battle! now go!
Swiftly sapped, my strength again,
To think and think again.
Far too much this task could be.
A day at a time too much?
Beware!

MAGICAL MINDS

DOWN AMONG THE DEAD MEN, THAT WAS ME
FOR MONTHS, NOT WEEKS, NOR DAYS
TABLETS TOOK, TO NO AVAIL, BLACK HOLE
COMETH.
ARMAGEDDON, I THOUGHT AND SOUGHT HIM
OUT
BOTTOM LINE I'M ON THE EDGE, IN A DAZE.
"RELAX, LET IT COME TO YOU, IT'S JUST A
PHASE" SAID HE
"RUBBISH" I SAID "IT'S MORE THAN THAT"
TAKE THESE TABLETS, THEY ARE GOOD FOR
YOU
OFF I TROT, PILLS IN HAND, HAPPY PILLS IN
HAND
TWO, FOUR, EIGHT WEEKS PASSED, WILL IT BE
MY LAST
SUPPLIES RAN LOW, I TOOK THEM LESS
WAY DOWN IN DARKNESS THAT WAS I.
THE SUN BEGAN TO RISE, OH YES, DARK
FOLLOWS LIGHT
I FORCED THROUGH ONCE MORE, FRESHNESS
CAME
TO BODY AND SOUL, SO NEAR YET SO FAR.
BI-POLAR, THE NAME OF THE GAME, ONE OF
THE SAME
POSITIVE-NEGATIVE, THEY MEET IN TIME, JUST
WAIT.
GOD HAD WAITED TOO LONG THIS TIME
ALCHEMIST TOLD, HE PUZZLED AND LOOKED
THEY TAKE YOU NOT TO THE DEPTHS OF HELL,

ON AND PAST YOU GO, ONE WAY TICKETS, NO
MORE
DARKEST DEPTHS OF LIVING DEATH, PURE
HELL
ON AND ON THEY TAKE YOU THROUGH
OF YES! IT'S TRUE

ME AND MY DOG

Come on pal let's have a run

Over the fields and far away

Bridges, ditches, over farm gates

Have a sit, smoke, watch the day,

Off again, a rabbit to chase

But he's too fast unlike my dog

Another dog? One to face

Up the hills, through the dales

Another stop to look around

Sun still shining, fields abound

Round we turn homeward bound

In back door, don't wake a soul

Our feet are black as coal

Clean up, wash and brush now back at home.

MIND HOW YOU GO

Mind how you go
You can then grow – a lot
Find yourself a seat or a slot
Relax – Go with the flow
Sit, think, positive thoughts
Comfortable? Let them go
The demons will stay away
Keep thinking good thoughts
The devils will stay at bay
And hopefully go away
Just relax, worry not
Cool as ice – not he, he's hot,
Hot as Hell.

MIND OF MY PEACE

Eternal unrest, rotting and foul, now trapped behind
the door,
This shining light with golden wings beheld my broken
soul,
Pain and suffering eased somewhat and goals were
set for me.
I grasped the sword, a grip so firm,
The stone gave up the blade.
Achievement came in many ways, my mind set on my
tasks,
'Twas for ME! It had to be, if I were to last the course,
A warden of the mind I have, a sister to guide my
way.

The lamp of life is in her hand an aid to tend her flock.
T.L.C. to comfort me, the wind beneath my wings,
The fight goes on: - so hard it's been, a miracle for sure
Thank God, I lost and found my MIND my future's now secure

MINDS EYE

Look, look into my eyes
Blood shot and red, sore as hell.
So much has been seen
In the eyes of my mind
None can see into the mind's eye
Only me, me for all I'm worth
Darkest demons, elation so high
That's a demon too, trust me
Down in the dumps, high as a kite
Torn in half it has some bite
Even now! Level too
Gives one a good life
Away from my mind's eye
Can now relax, to the day I die.

MORNING

Time and tide wait for no man
It's plain to see
Morning, noon and night
For all to see
Dusk, dawn morning
For all to see
Red skies night and day
For all to see
Man cannot defeat
That's plain to see
Nature rules the days
To see it's plain
Spring, summer
Autumn, winter
So watch, dear man
Mother Nature
Cannot be rushed
That's for all to see
That includes – you!

MY WAY

Sorry folks but I had to beat it my way,
No more stopping me in my stride,
I had to do it, to survive.
Go for it that's the word.
Defeat the feelings within.
All the way, I had to go,
That's hard but I knew I would win.
God told me you see!
Patience, dark follows light
Light follows dark
Just wait, see it through!

NATURE RULES THE WAYS!

BUDS IN MAY OF CROCUS GROWS
GREEN GRASS SHEDS WINTER'S GLOOM
MORNING SUN, THE COCKEREL CROWS
BIRDS NESTLE IN AND MAKE SOME ROOM,
FOR EGGS, AS SPRING TIME NOW ARRIVES
TREES, ALL BARE, NOW FACE THE SUN
ANIMALS SNIFF THE AIR, AND BADGER, HE
SURVIVES.
FROSTY MORNS STILL MAKE THEM RUN,
THE NIGHTS ARE LIGHTER NOW,
MOON AND STARS IN CLEARER SKIES
GIVE ALL A LOVELY SHOW
AND MAN? HE SITS AND SIGHS
IS IT HE WHO IS SO WISE?
YOU SEE IT, NATURE RULES AND HOW!

NO CAN DO!

Oh woe is me, I cannot pen an ode,
Can't seem to write at all
Perhaps I'm on the wrong road
I sit, and try, to no avail
My talent has left my abode
Cannot do a thing
My pen's run dry
It's enough to make me cry.
Boo Hoo!. So sad.

NUMB-ERS

I'm stunned, in shock, my mind is numb,
Two fold problems, I know not how
To deal with, or even forget
"One", it makes me angry, irate too!
T'other, sadness, disappointed, way down low,
I'm up to here with number "one!"
Total infringement, I feel it's touched,
The need to speak, or just carry on,
Is hard for me to choose
T'other now, has cut me down,
I can do no more, I'm split in half.
A little rest, clear my head,
I'll stand aside once more
Your champion!
One day though, my dear,
I'll stay down, but you know that
Assistance though with "One's" loose tongue,
He's hurt me more than t'other has or can,
Please fight my corner this one time,
I know not how to deal please!

OFF AND ON

One day I am off
Another I'm on

Then I've gone

Never are the days the same

One day I'm bright,

Next I'd be dim

Never the twain shall meet

One day I'm up

Then I go down

You say left

You say right

Cannot stay still a mo

To stay in the middle

Has a sense of fun

Makes me laugh and tiddle.

OLD ARTHUR

OLD ARTHUR WAS A JOLLY CHAP
HE WOULD OFTEN STOP AND HAVE A CHAT
EVERY DAY I PASSED HIM BY
HELLO GOOD CHEER, HE'D CALL OUT
THURSDAY LAST OLD ARTHUR CAME
AND CHATTED AND LAUGHED AWHILE
NEXT DAY, NO ARTHUR, WHERE'S HE GONE
MRS. MAY, SHE CALLED ACROSS
HE DIED LAST WEDNESDAY EVE
WELL WHO'D I SEEN ON THURSDAY LAST
A SPIRIT, A GHOST, HE NEVER WENT PAST.

OLD SHINER

The man in the moon, a happy soul,
His rays so bright at night
A man from earth once stood his ground
On the crust of planet moon
He stayed a while and off he flew
To earth to look again
So bright now shone the orb so high
'Twas dark and cold up there
No heat, dust and craters abound
Down here a warm glow shines
Alights our paths as we travel on
Until the dawn does break.

ON THE MEND

On the mend, that's me!
Bad thoughts, highs and lows
Seem to be drifting out to sea
And every door they close
No allowance to return
Hell for them to burn, forever
Eternal peace is mine
Must retain it, that's clever!
I'll not cry, I'll not pine
The universe is mine, forever.

ONE WAY TICKET

"YOUR COUNTRY NEEDS YOU" THE POSTER
SAID.
THREE SONS, SO YOUNG, TOO YOUNG TO DIE.
BROTHERS THREE, NOW EIGHTEEN?
THEY SIGNED THE FORMS, ALL LIED OF
COURSE.
DEATH WARRANTS THEY WERE,
BUT PRIDE AND GLORY OVERCAME.
AS FIGHTING MEN THEY MARCHED TO HELL.
THEY LAUGHED AND JOKED, WAR GAMES TO
PLAY.
THE KILLING FIELDS AWAIT
AND THE POPPY'S RED GLOW BECKONS.
MUD AND BLOOD TOGETHER RAN
TANKS, CANNONS, GUNS
BAYONETS TOO! CRASHED ALL ABOUT,
THE BOYS NOW FEARED THE WORST.
THREE DAYS IT TOOK THE BOYS TO DIE
PARENTS FEARS NOW FOUNDED
NO MORE THEY LAUGHED
JUST TEARS FOR THEM
THREE BABES NOW IN THE GRAVE
ONE WAY TICKETS ALL POSSESSED
LITTLE DID THEY KNOW
SNATCHED FROM US SO YOUNG, SO BRAVE
LIKE AUTUMN LEAVES THEY DROPPED, BLOWN
AWAY FOREVER.
THOSE MUDDY TRENCHES CLAIMED THEIR
SOULS.
REMEMBER THEM, IN YOUR HEARTS,
THEY DID NOT DIE ALONE.

OVERLOAD

Tell them all to take it slow,
Too fast will let you down
Stress will creep upon your soul
It's seeking to destroy
Marriage, Health, your very life
The lot, if you're not cautious
Enjoy yourself, eat good food
And moderate your work or else.
The weight of the world becomes you,
With worry and fatigue, no less
Have a drink, perhaps three or more,
To relax you'll pop a pill,
Until such time it's catch 22
And you are in the shit,
Fear not, life's a beach, enjoy it now,
You'll be a long time gone,
Look to boundaries and you must keep,
It's survival of the fittest.

PASS TOO SOON

TENDER TEARS FOR FRIENDS NOW PASSED
TENDER TEARS FOR THEY MAYBE YOUR LAST
WE'VE LOST THEM OLD TOO OFTEN YOUNG
THE BEST HAVE LEFT US, UNSUNG.
NO FIGHTERS HERE, NOR HEROES THERE
JUST THE COMMON PEOPLE TO STOP AND
STARE
HERE ONE DAY GONE THE NEXT
OUR HEARTS ARE TORN TO SHREDS
READ THE OLD, THE NEW, IT'S ALL THE SAME,
PASSING FRIENDS PASS TOO SOON.

PEACE IN ETERNITY

Burning candle, sharp and bright
I see the light, it burns.
Take me forward, that's right
Can see it all, even terms
To help me from my Hell
I have a tale to tell
From Hell to Utopia
My mind is clear
Must do this talk
Advance, advance no fear
Must go quick and fast
Then forever I will last
"Eternity!"

PEACE OF MY MIND

'Twas time to go, the time had come,
The scenic roller coaster slows,
Twists and turns, ups and downs: - too much!
Crash! Off the rails, to peace perhaps?
Trauma tears my mind to shreds, unseen.
Move to end the pain, I say!
Toxins flood painlessly, submission from the soul.
In a shaft of light, I came to Mind,
At peace and not alone, protected and so safe,
Hands came forth and shadows moved to help me
swim ashore,
One stood bold, a shaft of light, the saviour shone so
bright,
A bond had formed; unique it is to this very day.
Evil taunts of old, so bad, fade and vanish in the
glare.

PEACEHAVEN SANCTUARY

Man or woman
Male or female
It's hard to know who's who.
A man skin deep
Female within
Crying to escape, be free!
Understanding? – "queers and poofs!"
That's man's equation of this
Freak of Nature, no more, that's all,
Support is all they ask
Imagine if you will – read on,
Joint feelings in your mind;
A reject of the soul.
Courage bids to win through,
So be proud to reach your goal,
Now rest and enjoy your lot.
In peace!

PIECE WORK

A few minders came upon a hill
Atop was sanctuary – high aloft
Too high, perhaps for just so few
Blood, sweat, tears and skill
The going would be hard, not soft.
Archers lifted their bows so high
To break the nearer ground
Volunteer troops too, must aim for the sky
To reach the ultimate goal
Peacehaven they had within their grasp
They settled there a while or two
Serenity would be a hard nut to crack
Moneylenders were sought to woo
We gained this for food and arms
Settled once more, many had left
The cash flowed in dribs and drabs
"Go with the flow" – St. Teresa said
They hailed and looked about
We have our wizards and our wands
"Let's cast a spell, right now", the archers cried
Fund raisers, fire raisers, all must work so hard
Just to gain a sanctuary with aces high the card
Time will come for battle to cease
So's all can rest their weary piece.

POOR DANNY

Where's my mate gone, old Dan
Saw him on Tuesday, now they say he's dead
Can't be, not Dan, he's a wily fox.
Saw him Wednesday, he's ok, told me so,
Saturday sees him dead, poor soul.
He phoned me on Friday, to wish me ok.
Heard no more till Monday eve,
When a knock upon the door told all
Dan's been found, upon his chair and affront of TV
screen
Stone cold poor Dan, old Dan, friends forever.

POTATO CRISPS

Yum, yum, munchy stuff

These crisps they are so good.

Munch Munch!, the pack has gone

Another one bites the dust

I feel full up, but don't give up.

They make you smile, they make you cry

Sometimes they make you sigh

These elusive crunch crisps.

Walkers of course!

PRAISE BE

Praise be – The Lord is following me
Step by step – two by two
Walking close, without a shoe
He looks out in times of woe
To make sure I'm ok
Home or away, always there, unseen
I feel he's there behind me
Watching my every move
Left, Right, up or down, he knows where
More than I do sometimes
Praise is! No footprints in the sand
Just a presence of mind.

R.I.P.

The Angel of the Lord came down
To help a hollow soul
Devil had played a game or two
On this soul upon his knees
To this also the devil sent games
And did crack souls mind
The angel raised his arms
The soul did rise and rise
To heaven and eternal life.

RETURN FROM HELLSTAR

My dearest friends, supporters too!
The tales are nearly done, oh yes!
Journey back was not clear though
'Twas harder than I thought
As I sped, so fast, to Peacehaven
Realisation and logic return together,
I even thought I controlled the weather
Years flooded past, the blasted lot,
I cried and pinched myself
Too many good signs, so powerful,
'Twas my own sound barrier
Only a one way ticket now
To mother earth, her bosom warm
But signs still perceived
Logical now, I'd almost forgot!
I panicked to keep my wits
The demons waved to me so far,
And said clear off, you get on our tits!
We're staying here in hell
El-Tel!
A star with wings too!

RETURN TO EDEN

Man's way is not the way
Destruction, famine and war
Personal millions so many have
Most have none at all – zero
When will the meek inherit the earth?
Soon, don't worry, you'll see it soon
Nature wins through, our man is lost
Mother earth, valiant at no cast
The universe survives forever
Eden returns in clover – indeed.

RIPPERS TALE

Oh yes! It's me! Jack the Ripper.
Out of sight I come out at night
Knife and bag in hand
Ready for the first whore
To slice and cut at will.
I'll jump out and pull her to the floor
Hand over mouth, I'll slit.....
Her cool white neck, that's it
Then I'll open her up
To remove, and place in a cup
"My trophy, success"
Another one bites the dust
More to come? That's your guess
Oh yes it satisfies my lust.

RODENTS EAR!

Beware, beware, you had better believe!
I'm back, yes me, strong as a lion!
Fifteen years of Hell – pure Hell,
Resting now, with thoughts abounding,
My sword in scabbard tight,
Peace! Rest awhile, that'll do,
Journey's been so hard and long,
Harder than a diamond gem,
Blacker than the blackest coal,
Stuck in that bloody hole,
Diamond clear my mind will be,
Prize-fighter, that's me, a life, that's what I've won!
Remember too -
You ain't seen nothing yet!
My fighting days are done!
My pen is mightier than my sword.

RUN AGROUND

HI, HO, IT'S ME THE MAN WITH SONG
HI, HO, THE MAN WHO CANNOT SMILE
HI NO, HE'S DONE NO WRONG
HI, HO, HE'S NOT SMILED FOR A WHILE
WHAT'S WRONG? YOU ARE A HAPPY SOUL
A FIRE CRACKER AT A DO!
NO MORE TO LAUGH AND SING
'TWAS DEEMED TO BE A SIN
"NO" SAID THE LORD, "YES" SAID THE DEVIL
YOU KNOW NOT WHAT WAY TO TURN
STICK WITH THE LORD, HE IS THE HUB
TO TURN YOUR LIFE AROUND
AND SAVE YOU FROM RUNNING AGROUND.

SEAWAY TO HEAVEN
NO WAY BACK

I ran across the beach so far,
Until I reached the mud,
This surface was more a swamp,
It sucked and drew me in
What ere I did, it pulled me down
Into the slimy stinking mass
My grave, my resting place, I thought,
Was this to be my end?
Up to chest, my breathing tight,
I struggled without success
An hour passed, I had not moved,
But slipped a foot or more.
My arms now gone, I moved too much,
Sand to past my beard
Oozing through my open mouth
I screamed and screamed again
Blinded by black slime and mud
My body surrendered its soul
Down, Down, one way now
To death and heaven's gates.

SEE THE LIGHT

I LOOK UP AND SEE THE LIGHT.
I LOOK DOWN AND SEE THE SHADE.
LIGHTNESS AND DARKNESS, HIGHS AND LOWS,
THAT'S ME MOST OF THE TIME.
UP AND DOWN IN MY MIND.
UPS ARE EXHILARATING,
DOWNS ARE HELL.
I HAVE MANY GUARDIAN ANGELS
FAMILY, FRIENDS, PETS EVEN.
THEY ARE ALL MY FRIENDS.
AND THEY HAVE SAVED ME,
ONCE, TWICE OR EVEN THRICE,
AND REMEMBER READER,
A MAN WHO HAS FRIENDS CANNOT BE A
FAILURE.

SEEKING SANCTUARY

A pair we've been for 30 years
Ups and downs we've had a few.
Come through each and every one
The godsend was the care for me
As if struck by a mortal wound
Once carers came in force to me
We carried on our task
Our love, house and family
All remained intact – friends too!
More relaxed we have to be,
Perhaps I'll write a book
We'll see.

SEESAW

Up and down, that's me, a seesaw
Can't get off too easy
Feel sick – no way out
Life's a bitch, to the core
It seems I'm here forever
The duration – Eternity – no more
Better be here than in hell
Yes I'd rather be here oh yes!
God keeps me going that's for sure
My mind is not my own
Up and down, up and down, up and down
Oh dear, I cannot take much more
Wish it would burn out or snap
It does! For a time, not long
I'll have to learn to live with it
Oh no I'll not, you've got it wrong
Living's not easy, but I'll cope
Watch it demons of the mind
It's your swansong.

SHE MAN

God sent his daughters down
Not for one and all to see
As Jesus was, he paid the price
His daughters returned and said their bit
The lord heeded and pondered awhile
Standing up – he's made up his mind
Tears ran down his cheeks
"I'll go from here to create again
A being so meek and mild!
"How?" said sons, daughters and angels too
"Gender is the problem here – I'll solve it at a stroke
Bear children now my ladies dear
For all shall be as one, the same"
A freak they say – how dare they!
To save the earth the Lord united man and woman as
one
"Where did you get that idea?" they cried
"From St. Teresa" he said, and left forever
The earth grew as he wished
And heaven combined with earth
Eternal life in Eden once more
Believe me, that's for sure
Nostradamus, major powers, conflict will fail
Devils deeds will come to now't
The Lord has written on a stone
""Tis Peacehaven now – for eternity"

SHOW ME THE WAY

Can anyone show me the way?
I'm lost and have been for years
Please help me dear God
I stumble as I go, here and there
I cannot see the way
To settle and relax, it's easy
So they say, yes, no!
Ying Yang, a balancing act
For me to try, I hope
Maybe make it undo
So that I can see
And walk in a straight line
For all to see
It's been a long time
For one to be lost
Times gone by, that's it
"Maybe so my son"
Says the Lord
"But I've walked with you all the way"

SINGLE RAIL

I walk a double track
One up, one down
Black hole to supreme elation
As low as high, don't frown
Maybe I'll never come back
On a journey no one wants
I have to venture, no choice!
Keeps me going, one voice
Highs and lows all bad
Keeps me going, one voice
A voice of hope, no more
Try it and see, think positive
Yes it works for all to see
Perhaps now, we'll stop for tea.

SLAUGHTER OF THE INNOCENTS

One moment children's laughter,
Was heard to fill the air,
Then suddenly their living ceased,
Came nothing but despair.
He strode with guns-a-blazing,
Holding murder in his eyes,
And deadly bent on vengeance

SLUMBERING TIDE

The shingle is cast across the beach
Tide rises and ebbs so gently
A man lies upon the sand
In a deep sleep he lies
Tide rises and lifts him away
Floating out to sea,
He stays prone as if dead
Float, float, as far as ones eye can see.
Daylight, darkness, daylight again,
Tide flows in with man afloat
Still prone as if asleep
He would have known where the tide goes
Had he not been asleep, like Bo Peep.

SOLDIERS WENT

Soldiers went to places of hope
Foreign parts, hot and cold
Fighting, killing, will they cope?
What for? One asks!
See Bush or Blair for a dope
Who sent us here to the right of the line
Killing fields, our work is done
Fly home to family
Some were in pieces, some not
Others, torn to shreds, remain
No hero's welcome just a wave
Heads done for killings done
It'll be in one's mind forever
Sorry, but thy will be done.

SPARTAN WARRIORS

LIKE LIGHTENING, THEY CAME,
SWORDS AND GUNS IN HAND
HORSES STEAMING ON THE SNOW
CHILDREN, WOMEN, THEY FLED FROM THIS
HUNTING FOOD THE BRAVES HAD GONE
DECAPITATION! BLOOD RUNS FREE
UNARMED THEY BE, NO ARMS TO CALL,
SWARMING SOLDIERS, STING LIKE BEES.
KILL THE TRIBES, NO INDIAN FREE
THIS PLACE, OF COURSE, WOUNDED KNEE!
"PEACE ON EARTH AND GOODWILL TO ALL
MEN".

SPENT FORCE

A hill to climb, another one
Though not too bad nowadays
'Twas mountains that did test my grit
I wanted to jump, God held me back
"Hell awaits those who do!" he said
I cried and screamed to clear my mind
Alone with this I was, oh yes!
Doctors came and went, no more
They hardly had a clue
Another job, a pill or two
You're spaced out, the world unreal
It's time to tie the knot
You swing, expire, all the help around
Surgery to legs and arms, hearts and kidneys too,
In the mind, no knife can go.
Experiments are few
Sane or insane? A thin line here
It can come to one and all.
For me, I feel I've had my fill
And would like to terminate.
No more to climb and climb again,
To rest and drop out to relax
Livings too much for me at times
Achievements now have worn so thin.
"What's the point?" I ask
I get up – do – and go to bed,
Home or away its the same to me.
I'm bored beyond belief.
To get involved and work again
Would see me back on "10"
No, that's not for me, I'd rather die.
Pray God I do. And soon!

SPIRIT IN THE SKY

Religion is no cross or church
Green pastures, fresh air, the autumn leaves
The blowing of the winds, as seasons roll.
Man created none of these, he seeks now to destroy
Nature's way will win the day; the meek will stand so
proud.
Guardian angels all around, no wings or halos seen.
They work, heads down, knowingly of course
Material items has no time, oh no!
The earth will repair the damage done
And we will return to Eden (paradise)
Pollution gone, its bubble burst,
No fossil fuels – all gone
The power of earth, wind and rain,
Is everlasting. You'll see.

SPIRITUAL BONDS

Friendship, a gift of the gods,
A bond, so easily broken or lost.
One word can wash it away.
Not ours, OH NO! It's heaven sent.
As mother earth regains her strength.
She smiles at our six souls,
Our bodies purely lent to us,
To see us through this life.
Miles apart, we think as one,
Some may not agree.
But when we meet, the warmth within,
Goes through us all, as one, you see!

SPIT-FIRE AND HURRICANE

Calm and settled was the land
The skies a cloud or two.
Spit-fire came and screamed at foe,
Over horizon they showed their face
Dog and cat fury fought
Victory was to be had
To lose was not a thought
Spit-fire became too strong for all
Hurricane joined the fray
Stole spit-fire's thunder as all did fall
A tiger in his tank
When spit-fire screamed
Old hurricane roared
Sortie done? – They calmed and flew together.
United.
1936-45.

SUN D'RISE

The flower in bud
Bees in their drones
Drying up, that's the mud
Birds sing in tones
Tortoise lifts his head
From his cosy bed
A piece of lettuce for him
Because he likes it
Grass grows ready for a trim
Prepare garden and sit
To enjoy the rest away you're days
Sun so bright, skies so clear
It shines and beams as one lays
Asleep, of course, all day

SWEET REVENGE

I'VE BEEN TO HELL SO MANY TIMES
NEVER HAVE I BEEN BURNT – OH NO!
I WAS NOT ALONE ON THE JOURNEY – MAN
FOUR FOLLOWED ME THROUGH THE ABYSS –
OH YES!
JULIE, KEVIN, STEVEN – JEANNEY TOO FORGET
NOT J.C.!
THEY HOPED ME THROUGH THIS RING OF FIRE
I NEVER SAID THIS BEFORE
COULDN'T SEE THE POINT, YOU SEE
TO ME LIFE IS JUST A BORE
THE END WAS SWEET REVENGE, YOU SEE
DEVILS, DEMONS, TEMPTATIONS TOO
WERE LAID AT MY DOORWAY
TO THOSE I WAS ILL AND POORLY
DEATH WAS NOT A LOSS – I COULD NOT GIVE A
TOSS
MY ARMY CAME THROUGH FOR ME, SO
STRONG
TO TRUST IN GOD WAS IN MY MIND
MANY DID NOT KNOW THAT, SO SAD,
TIMES I COULD COPE, WITH LOTS OF HOPE
VICTORY, DEFEAT, I FELT SO GLAD
I WAS READY TO DO DEEDS AGAIN
THOUGH NOT WITHOUT MY TRUSTY CLAN
ALL BATTLES WOULD BE LOST
HARD AS NAILS THAT'S ME
HOLD YOUR BREATH, WAIT AND SEE
FOR ALL YOU'LL SEE IS ME
I'D DO IT ALL AGAIN – FOR THEM
ALIVE, ALIVE! THAT'S A GEM
YOU SEE IT'S ONLY ME, HAVE A NICE DAY.

SWEETHEARTS

Alone was I – A rebel too!
I hunted with the hounds,
Crowd a many – down to two,
Both bachelors for life, we thought?
One eve we met, I took to her,
Her Dad was a friend indeed,
Football supporting was his game,
A journey to a football match, ensured our path way
laid,
I put no plans or thoughts to her,
We took all within our stride,
A fireman now, we got on well,
Time to plan ahead.
June it was, a bond was formed,
United in our goal,
October 5th, West Ham drew,
We met the crowds, they cheered.
A party held with all our folk.
To leave at 9, we had to go
Car and train await, to Saltdean,
Our honeymoon does start,
Looking back o'er thirty years, three children,
Three moves to make a better place,
To settle and relax, retire,
Sit back you pair and look around,
Who could have done it better?
No one!

SWEETS

The sweets are on the side for me,
The sweets on the side are for me,
A dish, a dish full of joy
I'm glad I'm such a little boy!
Hungry for love and T.L.C.
Cry out loud and cry some more
Let's have them for tea!
Marshmallows, Jelly babies – Corr!
Munch, Munch, I'll eat the lot
Now for a sleep upon my cot
To dream sweet dreams
Night Night, God Bless.

TALK

Do you know what it's like?
When your enemy wins and wins.
You can't, it's impossible
For some, maybe, - not me.
Go for it, fight the evil within
In, through and out of hell's hole
I want my life back,
Not on the bloody rack
Know how to do it, I do!
Put some fun back in your life
Talk to a listener
Talk the demons out.

TEL'S REWARD

The Lord summoned El Tel
He'd done him proud
Fighting under a spell
"What worldly goods can I endow?"
El Tel said he wanted none
My life has taken away some twenty years
You owe me that at least
My career, jobs, nearly my marriage – all gone
I should feel anger for you God
You've put me through black hell
I then came back, from where no man can tell
You owe me Lord, ruler of all
I could have got more from Solomon and Saul
Peace and serenity, I wish to be granted
To re-build my life, maybe too late
I'll not come home yet, so shut the gate, he did,
On his way out!

TENDERFOOT GEORGE

A friend we lost, so suddenly,
A brother, taunted by the past,
The horrors of darkness, loneliness too,
With flowing locks and denim cloth
He strove for peace and freedom,
In god he trusted, his spirits strong,
He loved; - a shaft of light to his soul,
A troubled soul, now shattered and torn
"Hello" a smile, to all he met,
His faith intact, he fought alone,
"Little Big Horn" – his battle won.
"Wounded Knee" warriors end,
He too, alas, could fight no more,
His scars and wounds so very deep.
The doves, they called him to rest,
Too much; - too long; - come now
The owl had called his name
He sang no more for us to hear,
Like autumn leaves blown softly away.
To rest in peace: - "A spirit in the sky!"
Love me tender forever more. Amen.

THE BULLDOG BREED?

British is best, that's what they say,
Our cars are made abroad,
Mines are shut and sealed,
Beef is best, oh, not it's not!
B.S.A, Norton, Triumph too
Motor bikes are dead and gone.
Old Honda saw to that,
Football, cricket, rugby too,
All take us on – and win.
Electronics, the Japs can do,
So please John Bull, what is best?
I cannot fathom out!

THE CLEANING MAN

Buckets, cloths and mops
In and out I slop
Wipe here, wipe there
Never miss a bit
Busying along without a care
I hardly have time for a sit
Leathers for windows
Mops for floors
Rub the dirt till it goes
Keep your hands off, mucky paws,
I have my pride
And that's for me to ride
Cos I'm the cleaning man
Name's Dan ok!

THE FINAL RUN

CAMPBELL PERISHED ON CONISTON,
BLUEBIRD LIFTED, TURNED AND SANK.
'TWAS THE CALMEST DAY SO FAR
CARCASS LOST, HIS SOUL LONG GONE,
NOW LOOK ACROSS THE LAKE – SO WIDE,
IT'S MYSTERY HELD – DEEP DOWN,
IN FATHOMS OF CONSITON WATER – NOW –
REVEALS A CHILL OF TIMES PAST,
WHEN CAMPBELL RACED HIS CRAFT,
BACK AND FORTH – HIS DESTINY DUE
THE EDGE WAS NEAR, TOO FAR, HE WENT,
HIS FATHER DID THIS TOO,
"SPEED KILLS!" IT DID FOR THEM
THE HEROES IN OUR HEARTS!
R.I.P.

THE FIREBRAVES – ULTIMATE SACRIFICE

The call sounds for all to hear
All heed and run to help
Fire, crash, persons trapped, who knows?
They slip into their gear, no fear
Engines start, on they climb
Opening doors unleash these braves
They go to a fate unknown
Explosions heard, they near their goal,
A fireball lights the sky
Turning wheels, the scene is seen
Two have jumped, one is trapped
Two braves don breathing sets
Into hell they go to seek
Infernos child cannot be found
A cry "back room" is heard by both
They turn and hear a child
Leader in he slips and falls
The raging fire strengthens
From a gap in smoke a child is plucked
From hell to mother's arms
Alive he is for all to see
Fallen hero still inside
A crew is called and in they go
Too late, this now, explosion two
Rips heart and soul from all
Down to earth this job brings them
Their colleague is no more
50/50 that's the chance
The child lived and grew a man
The brave, he died, an angel now
A guardian for his kind

THE LIGHT

The light, the light
I see the light,
Now maybe I'm saved
From the awful illness
Maybe manic has caved
I can't stand much more
It's too much for any man
I want to love and caress
To be "normal" whatever that is
See the world again, happily
For me to see the light
It may give me a fright
Already has! It's time to grow
Achieve now all you've wished
Go for it Tel boy, you can do it
If you do, well you'll excel.

THE "MIND" HEALER

WHAT NEED OF WEALTH? MATERIALISTIC GAIN
IS NOTHING MORE TO ME AND DOES NOT
PLEASE
NOR SATISFY MY AIM WHEN ALL AROUND
I MAY OBSERVE A FELLOW MAN IN GRIEF
I SEEK NO PRAISE TO LEND A WILLING HAND
TO HELP A FALLEN COMRADE TO RISE AGAIN
AND IF A MOMENT OF MY TIME BE SPARED
A LISTENING EAR MIGHT EASE A HEART IN PAIN.

EACH TENDER WORD OF COMFORT MIGHT
ENDURE
LONG AFTER TEARS OF SORROW HAVE BEEN
SHED
IF ANY ACT, OR SOUND, OR WRITTEN DEED
CAN INSERT JOY INTO A LIFE THAT BLED
THROUGH AGES WITH REMORSE AND MISERY
THEN SPREAD THAT, WHICH MAY BRING A
CLEAR RELIEF,
AND KNOW THAT ANY FORM OF LOVE WHEN
GIVEN
WILL FLOURISH IN ITS GROWTH OF PURE
BELIEF.

HE WHO WALKS WITH HIGH UNDAUNTED
COURAGE
AND HIDES NOT HIS HUMILITY TO MAN,
WHO SHOWS TO ALL HIS GLORIOUS
COMPASSION
IS EVEN CONSCIOUS OF HIS FATHER'S PLAN.

THE UGLY DUCKLING

I've a mind, to let it grow,
So big to surely glow
Small acorn, it was when we arrived
We strived to make it great
Help line, Counselling, with training too!
We began to make our mark
Into. Line our lodge so large
For members all, the meek and mild
Of troubled minds and souls
Lady Archer stood over all
To see we got it right.
She smiled and laughed throughout our task
Money came, wizard saw to that
A shop, a shop, my kingdom for a shop
Was the loudest cry
Property gained, furnished too
A mind shop for me and you
Volunteers came and got a job
To serve and carry for one and all
Time rolled on and budget swelled
"Give us a sanctuary!" cried one lost soul
A halfway house would fit the bill
We begged and borrowed, asked Branson too
To fulfil our dream, sanctuary!
In 2006 the lights went on
Our task was now complete
Well, we knew we could not be beat!
Our ugly duckling was now a swan.

THE VOLCANO – OR IS IT ME?

Hubble bubble, toil and trouble
I had lain dormant for years
Then I erupt for one and all
"Run, run, let us flee" is the call
I rumble and blast for all my peers
Liquid flows, Etna is manic
High as a kite she goes
Only to settle and rest
So slow, she sleeps and retires
Till the next time
After she's settled to rise again oh yes.

THE WINDOWS OF MY MIND

Can you see through?
The windows of my mind
Sometimes bright and clear
Others dark and grimy
Blimey! That sounds grim
Can't see for the dust
When bright and clear it's great
Life's a beach, oh yes!
When dark, life's a bitch
So help me God, where's the duster?

THEY COULD NOT WIN

Traders came and killed the herds,
Land and gold attracted more,
Railways cut through holy shrines,
Fortresses and soldiers came,
To hunt and kill the tribes,
Treaties made and broken.
Land and rivers grabbed from them,
No buffalo now roam the plains,
No clothing, food and rivers foul,
The heart ripped out of them.
Soldiers lived by guns and swords,
Greed and corruption fired them on.
Rights? We have none
"The only good Indian is a dead one!"
They said in Washington's Halls.
'Tis now, today, they sit on land
And think upon the past.
Reservations, that's their homes,
Their spirits still intact.
One day, white man, we will see you done,
Nature's way will tell – and win!

TOO MUCH TO LOSE

The way is there, my Peacehaven,
Its loss would be too much,
From this place, my life was saved
And changed, enriched, forever more.
In our fleet it stands alone,
Within range and sights of foe,
Lack of funds will start her slide,
We'll lose the bloody lot.
From two well meaning listening ears,
A dozen now, to support and aide.
We must not lose my Peacehaven
I'll never feel the same, oh no!
Valerie Lodge, Southernay – havens not for me.
Peacehaven is my ship; so safe!
So far; so long, its been second home to all
Just for me, save my ship and
I can remain forever more.

TOO TIRED FOR FIGHTING

My back was bent, my hands crooked
Too long had I fought, too long.
Not against a seeing thing
Something beyond the soul
Comes at you from a black hole
Can't be seen, nor a scream
By God he goes in deep
What is it he wants?
This demon within
"You" is what he wants my son
Fight on and you will win
I will, I will, he's only skin deep.

THUNDER JACK

Thunder Jack was called to arms
Fire and water opposed him now
Not shields, not swords but lucky charms
Good fortune he would need; and how!
Twenty years he fought the might
Of fire, despair and grief
Depression, not a word he saw in sight
Sadness, he watched it every day
Others losses mirrored on him
One day he'd have to pay
Carry and battle on, heeding not a whim
Lucky charms left one day, he did not have a say
Ladders crashed and left old Jack
A laying on the deck akin an empty sack
Struggled back, he toiled – in pain
Half the man he was, poor jack!
Too much now a tear would stain
Jack would ne'er give in
Oh no not he! A man of steel
His mind though, wasn't strong
His time was up, that made him reel
M.O. said "Right" Jack said "Wrong"
He turned and battled on.
Horrors came upon his mind
The power was now upon
Jack sobbed now and gave his axe
Up for all to see and sigh
Fear not dear Jack, your axe goes on
Young'uns come and bonds do tie
It'll not end when you're gone!
No fear.

TIME GENTLEMEN PLEASE

The earth does not belong to man
Man belongs to earth.
Humans will last no time at all.
Their damage will repair.
Mother earth saw seasons change
How could man alter that?
Man travels along, pollution in his wake,
Ignorance, malicious, gain, money,
Whatever the cause it needs redress.
Nature will clear the air, in time,
Dinosaurs once ruled the lands,
Man has taken too much now,
It's time to reclaim it all.
Iron Age, Ice Age, Stone Age, Human Age,
All will pass, to die, and wither,
The paradise age moves in.

TITANIC – COLD GRAVE

'Twas from afar the ice was seen
A cry below to all the crew
Crash and roar! The 'berg was through, clean!
Metal gaped, a hole clear through.
"She'll sail" they said, Lifeboats are few!
Passengers awoke, but turned and sighed.
Listing hard, now panic grew
Oh ship builders, have you lied?
"Unsinkable" they said to one and all
She'll sail no more over seas to rule.
Darkness came to all that night
Into the sea and out of sight.
Some boats saved to see the dawn
"Thank God", they said, and home to scorn!
The Titanic wasn't unsinkable.
Unthinkable! R.I.P.

TOTAL RECALL

IT'S MINE! TOTAL RECALL,
YOU'VE SEEN THE FILM
WELL THAT'S IT.
I'M BACK, 15 YEARS OF HELL,
I'M BACK, 15 YEARS OF PURGATORY
I'M BACK, WITH A VENGEANCE!
HELL THAT HATH NO FURY!
IT'S GONE – THANKS TO MIND!
NOW WE GO FORTH,
SWORDS IN HANDS,
PENS IN POCKETS
TO BEAT THE DEMON FACE
GREENPEACE, THAT'S THE ANSWER,
LET'S RID THE WORLD OF DRUGS, ABUSE
CRIME!
LET'S GO FOR IT – GREENPEACE.
SENT FROM ABOVE!
ABOUT TIME TOO!
LET'S DO IT.
NOW!
IF YOU'VE A MIND TOO!

TOUCHED BY THE BRUSH OF MADNESS

From behind they speak/creep up,
The horrors from within
A fear, a shiver, just a start,
Their fun can do you in.
Like maggots they gnaw into your mind
Their circus tricks abound
In and out evil tongues do dart
Amongst dark shadows of your kind.
Silence is weakness, they love a start
The thoughts are there - suicide!
My god, I can't do that!
To shun this gift of life itself
A sin beyond a rat.
The devil's brush can paint your mind
The Lord fights for the soul
Jump into hell, if you wish.
Wait! Hold fast; paradise is my goal!
Be gone foul painter in my head
I'll fight you till I'm dead
Demon brush and palette, now within my grasp.
For me to touch old Satan
Will turn madness into calm!
I behold his brush; no more to harm!
It's a question of balance, old man!

TREES 'A' GREEN 'TILL AUTUMN'S FALL

Teresa came, a while back now,
To mind that is: Peacehaven.
She grew so fast, and blossomed too!
No ugly duckling, but a swan, so proud.
Her phoenix had risen at last.
Future planned, and past at rest
Her winter became her spring, with us,
To toil and enrich our very souls,
An open book, she was a gem.
Family grown and raised so well
Her roots grew deep with Mind.
One in a billion you could say she was,
Perhaps we could all be that way?
A daily joy to see and work
Her aims were all for Mind, no doubt!
A golden heart she had, and it showed
A diamond within our crown,
Platinum soul, so sacred too,
She blessed all whom she met, so kind.
Dark clouds formed so fast they came.
A storm to destroy our "Trees".
She slipped away, no warning here,
You'll ne'er find a mind to match
Irreplaceable you see, oh yes!
"Go with the flow" she said to me,
And now of course she has.
On autumn's day, she drifted away
The sanctuary gates await, ajar
Trees now have golden leaves,
Teresa's found eternal peace

Serenity, that too, of course!
Bless her.

TWO FACES

WE HAVE TWO FACES, ALL OF US,
JECKYLL AND HYDE, THAT'S LIFE
NOT STRANGE, JUST LIFE, THINK ON!
A FACE FOR WORK, IT MUST IMPRESS
THE FACE FOR HOME, CAN DEPRESS.
TWO PEOPLE, ONE FOR HERE,
THE OTHER FOR ELSEWHERE.
ONE IS CALM AND PRETTY TOO.
T'OTHER IS ROUGH AND UGLY.
BOTH ALTHOUGH - ARE ONE!
CAN YOU BELIEVE IT, YOU'D BETTER,
NO EXCEPTIONS FROM THIS RULE.
DO WE REALLY KNOW OUR WIFE,
HUSBAND, BROTHER TOO!
PERHAPS WE FEEL WE DO!
WIN THE LOTTERY AND THEN WE'LL SEE,
THEN FRIENDS WILL DROP LIKE FLIES,
ENVY GREED AND FAMILY TOO,
WILL SNIFF AND WALK AWAY,
YOU CANNOT WIN, WHATEVER YOU DO!
WE CHANGE AS AGES PASS
WE ALL HAVE TWO FACES,
BELIEVE THAT OR GO ON YOUR WAY.

TWO MINDS

Retired now, it's time to write,
Rat race? No more for me,
It's too much for my mind,
Even up, relax, a coiled spring no more.
As I write, the music plays, memories abound
Tired now, I'll carry on, desk jobs that's for me.
I have to rest, for family's sake
Their plight was watching me.
Broken in a corner, half a man in tears.
That's at an end, I stand 6ft.
My back, it bends no more,
Paid work? No! leave me be,
I do no harm, I do my bit,
Quality of life, at last, don't touch!
Years of pain must not return.
No debts I owe to society.
My mind has seen to that.

TWO RED LIGHTS

ONLY TWO? THAT'S A JOKE
BLUE FLASHING ONES TELL THE TALE
EMERGENCY NO TIME TO STOP
HE'S REVVING UP SO FAST
STATUS QUO – HIS SPEED A TON,
HE'LL BURST AFORE HE DIES
HOLDING DOWN IS NOT THE WAY
SPEAK OUT AND GET SOME HELP.
IT'S IMPOSSIBLE ON HIS OWN
DOES HE REALISE, OH NO!
TELL HIM OFF AND SLOW HIM DOWN
HE'LL SETTLE IN THE DUST
"IF YER LUCKY" HE WILL SAY
THEN BURN AND BURN AND BURN
NOT DIE, JUST BURN, ON HIS KNEES
LET'S HELP HIM – PLEASE!

WATERWORLD

A car that runs on water?
Drugs that cannot kill?
Now that's a silly thought!
Chemicals no more – more herbal remedy?
Cancer, aids are gone from man
Plus drugs for a longer life
Now that's a silly thought!
Telecoms across the world, TV. Radio too?
Planes that fly over speeds of sound?
Now that's a silly thought!
No wars, just peace to see us through?
No battles like Bannockburn?
Now that's a silly thought!
Greenpeace fights for land and sea
The air I cannot see
Now that's a silly thought!
Animals not hunted for skins and decoration
Perhaps, one day, soon – God will have a coronation
Now that's a really silly thought
Green pastures, the Garden of Eden?
Walk naked, in the buff
Not me!
That is a silly thought
Money all gone, all is free
I've fallen from my tree
Now that's really stupid.

WHAT WAY

Oh Lord, what way now,
No more rocky roads with stones afoot,
No caverns with holes as black as hell,
Demons in my mind have ceased.
Only to return again so soon.
They carry no silver spoon,
Screaming Demons through my skull
From within my senses dull
Please oh Lord grant me this
A path so smooth and clear
Tell me that's the way to go
I can then go with the flow.

WHEN I FALL IN LOVE

When I fall in love, it will be forever,
When I give my heart, that's forever too!
Temptation, oh no! not ever, no way
I'll never fall in love again
Love is ended before it's begun
For me it's still forever
Always forever, no more
You can feel it so true
Eternity has started for you!

WHERE'S MY INSPIRATION GONE?

Where's my inspiration gone?
Where has it gone?
Could write two or three
Odes that is, poems too!
Pen in hand I sit, just me!
Sobbing and crying Boo Hoo!
I've got the lot – as you saw
No man could wish for more
Writer's cramp is that it?
Inspiration – It's gone hasn't it?
My mind seems empty to the core
Still, I'll sit here, still with pen in hand
Perhaps one day it will land
On me!

WHO?

Who? Yes who – is the wizard
Who? Sees one and all
Who? Saves one and all
Who? Sees the end of the world
Who does? Oh yes he does
Man's greed cannot go on
Our rivers must remain
Streams must run, with fish alive
Skies and clouds must remain – intact
Then we will see an Eden
Only then will we be happy – Who?

"WHY? – OH WHY?

IN '69, THE VICTIM FOUGHT,
YOUNG BOYS, AROUND 19, SO YOUNG,
"WHY?" WE ASKED, "THIS WAR TO FIGHT",
THEY SENT THEM ANYWAY.
VOLUNTEERS CAME AS NIXON CALLED,
ALL SIGNED AND SEALED THEIR FATE.
DEFEAT? THEY KNEW NOT WHAT THAT MEANT,
BOTH SIDES THAT IS, YES, BOTH.
MANY DIED, SOME STILL THERE,
THEY ROT IN STEAMING GLADES,
STOP, STOP, NO MORE TO DIE!
A FIGHT YOU CANNOT WIN,
MIGHTY MACHINES FLEW OVERHEAD,
ROTORS DRIPPING BLOOD,
STAINS REMAINED IN HANDS AND MINDS,
TRAUMAS OF THIS WAR,
VICTORY NOW, JUST A WORD,
ALL HAD DIED IN VAIN,
ENEMIES AWAIT THE ONSLAUGHT NOW,
BUT "HUEYS" RETURNED TO BASE,
TEENAGERS LEFT THAT FIGHT IN "NAM"
NOW THEIRS IS OVER HERE!
"WHY?" OH WHY?

WHY DO YOU SLEEP SO STILL?

Why and how do you sleep so sound?
Is it me or when I'm not around?
You snuggle up and off you go
It's only me who is so slow
I toss and turn, sweat up a bit
Early hours, they come and go
Still awake, and you snore in the pit
Why do you sleep so still?
Not a care in the world
You never take a pill
I'm up and down, you lay curled
Thoughts abound as I rest
As if I'm set a test.

WINDOWS OF MY MIND

The room, my room, pictures in array,
Memorabilia too! Vast amounts,
Of past and fondest interest,
Hang around these four walls.
In solitude I sit and write -
Listen, watch and relax
A world apart, no hurry, no worry,
My mind creaks – amidst this life,
It's seen too much, of blood and tears,
A bridge too far now burned to ash.
The future lies within these walls,
Books to pen and odes inspire,
With clearing mind, I commit to Mind;
My gateway for seven years.

WITCHES OF WHITMORE

MRS ARCHER SITS AT HER DESK
SHE WISHES SHE HAD SOME DOUGH
WORKING, WORKING, ALL THE WHILE
ALL WISH FOR BETTER TIMES, IN MIND OF
COURSE
YOU WOULD THINK SHE'D HAD ENOUGH
CASH! THAT'S WHAT YOU NEED!
SWAP IDEAS IN YOUR CAULDRONS NOW
THE WIZARD IS READY TO REVEAL
HE'S BOOKED YOU A PLACE IN HISTORY
SIT BACK MY ARCHER DEAR, RELAX
ALL WILL BE REVEALED
YOU'LL JUST HAVE TO BE PATIENT.

WORK NO MORE

I'll work no more
My mind is with Mind
To toil for them
It's easy you see
Make a cuppa
Give a smile
Answer door and phone
Archer keeps an eye
On me, she does
If I'm down I'm down
Mind lifts my heart
Supported I feel
Supported I am
Family and friends
One and all around
I'm the king
I've been crowned
That's how I feel
Thanks to my minders.

www.ingramcontent.com/pod-product-compliance
Lightning Source LLC
Chambersburg PA
CBHW031209270326
41931CB00006B/477